TRICK or TREAT

What your doctor isn't telling you about mood-altering medications.

Suka Chapel-Horst, RN, PhD, QMHP, CPLT

TRICK OR TREAT
What your doctor isn't telling you about
mood-altering medications.

Author: Suka Chapel-Horst, RN, PhD, QMHP. CPLT

Published by:
Brainworks Publishing
638 Spartanburg Highway, Suite #70-175
Hendersonville, NC 28792

www.IMRIWellness.org
www.AriseAlcoholRecovery.com

Neither the publisher nor the author is engaged in rendering professional advice or services to the individual reader. The ideas, procedures, and suggestions contained in this book are not intended as a substitute for consulting with your health care provider. All matters regarding your health require medical supervision. Neither the author nor the publisher shall be liable or responsible for any loss or damage allegedly arising from any information or suggestions in this book.

While the author has made every effort to provide accurate telephone numbers and Internet addresses at the time of publication, neither the publisher nor the author assumes any responsibility for errors, or for changes that occur after publication. Further, the publisher does not have any control over and does not assume any responsibility for author or third-party websites or their content.

ISBN-13 978-1494473952
ISBN-10 149447395X

ABOUT THE AUTHOR

I've had over forty years of experience as a Registered Nurse in the fields of mental health, criminal justice, addictions, and wellness education. I've worked in hospitals, addiction and detox centers, residential treatment centers for the mentally ill, residential homes for the mentally challenged, locked facilities and residential treatment homes for teenagers with criminal histories. I've been a jail nurse, home health nurse, operating room nurse, infertility education nurse, and owner of a nursing services business serving many residential treatment centers.

During this time I also attended a seminary program and was ordained as an inter-faith minister. This led to training as a hospital chaplain, and to becoming chaplain to a county sheriff's department. My doctorate is in religious studies and spiritual science.

My passion to teach and uplift comes from seeing so many people relapse, or get worse, despite years of counseling, therapy, and medications. I believed that there had to be a better way, a way that leads to healing and a good life.

Fortunately, over the years, I've been introduced to many alternative resources for recovery and to many healers, researchers, scientists, and leading-edge thinkers. We are in the forefront of a new and advanced approach to medicine and healing, bringing relief and an end to the needless suffering of so many, and I'm passionate about this.

May the information and resources offered in this Bottom Line Book be helpful and healing for you, and for your loved ones.

Books and DVDs by Dr. Suka Chapel-Horst

WORKBOOKS

How to Quit Drinking for Good and Feel Good

"Why Do I Feel This Way?" Natural Healing for Optimal Health and
> Relief from Moods and Depression

BOOKS

Take a Leap of Faith

DVD

Depression – Ten Different Sources / Ten Different Approaches
> Your Guide to Finding and Treating the Real Underlying Cause

BOTTOM LINE BOOKS

BOOKS/DVD PowerPoint Presentations

Wellness Simplified – How Food affects Moods, Bodies, and Behaviors

"Why Do I Feel This Way?" – Natural Healing for Optimal Health and Relief from Moods and Depression

PTSD – Alternative Resources for Recovery

The Real Cause and Solution for Alcohol Addiction

The Gift – A Sound Mind for Life

Cannabinoids: Marijuana, THC, CBN, Cannabis, CBD – The Hundredth Monkey Cure

These books and DVD's can be ordered through:
www.IMRIWellness.org
www.AriseAlcoholRecovery.com or by calling 417-380-3254

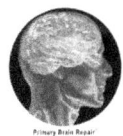

PRIMARY BRAIN REPAIR

Primary Brain Repair focuses on providing the brain, body, and spirit with the basic requirements for health and wellbeing. It's the first line response to all illnesses and disorders. It involves the use of natural micronutrients, nutrition therapy, exercise, and stress relief.

Optimal health can be achieved by most people by following these guidelines. For individuals who need more intensive treatment, these basic health steps will be the foundation that allows advanced treatment to be effective. When primary brain repair is not addressed, medications and counseling have little long-term effect.

Using simple, but effective, recovery tools, *Primary Brain Repair* will improve the health of everyone who applies it. How can that be? Simply, because we go back to the basics of how the brain and body are designed to work. The answer is in nature, and the method is natural.

At Integrative Memory Research Institute our mission and passion is to educate the public and healthcare professionals about the most advanced methods for obtaining optimal health, naturally. Based on the latest neuroscience and biochemical research, along with years of experience, Dr. Suka offers leading-edge knowledge and how-to information to those who are seeking real recovery versus symptom relief.

We are passionate about helping you. That's why we've created self-help books and DVDs to guide you through the process.

www.IMRIWellness.org
417-380-3254

INTRODUCTION

The pharmaceutical industry is a self-serving entity more interested in profit than the welfare of individuals in need of healing. With an unlimited ability to fund lobbying efforts in Washington, it controls legislative decisions as they relate to health and medicine. Proposals offered to government that support organic farming, natural foods and food supplements, have been denied or watered down due to pharmaceutical influence. The Food and Drug Administration (FDA) bows to "big pharma" in all decisions.

Investigative research is bringing to light the methods used by pharmaceutical companies to dupe the public. What we see and hear in promotional advertising is rarely the truth. These companies are not required to disclose privately owned research. Thus, only the studies that have had some, even a limited, degree of success are told.

Because negative side effects don't usually show up until after a few weeks, or months, testing stops short of the time when negative results might occur. Testing of drugs takes place in parts of the world that have no relationship to our foods or culture. Those being tested are often people in poverty, with little education, and are, therefore, unable to accurately report their reactions. The paid physicians who oversee the testing are encouraged to obtain positive results. And so on...

If one will take the time to check out specific medication descriptions, they will find that many clearly state, in my words, "we don't know how this drug works".

Robert Whitaker, in his eye-opening book, *The Anatomy of an Epidemic*, (2010, Crown Publishing Group) has researched the research and offers us a look at the intentional deception drug companies have used that allow for the numbing and dumbing-down of Americans as a result of the proliferation of mind and mood altering medications. Another excellent resource is *Overdo$ed America* by John Abramson, MD. (Harper Collins) I recommend reading these books if you are presently taking or considering the taking of any mood or mind altering medications.

As an RN in the mental health field for over forty-five years, I have seen the changes first hand and I find it frightening that so many Americans seem to be oblivious to the dangers and disastrous outcomes from long-term, chronic use of many medications.

I hope this Bottom Line Book will be enlightening to some and hopefully prevent actions that can lead to hopeless dead-end results. The very words, "you'll have to be on these medications for life" or "you should never stop taking your medications" only serves the drug industry.

It's time to put people first. That's you and I. This is a wake-up call. Please don't sleep through it.

My advice is to remain open to alternatives to traditional medical treatment. Seek out the natural resources that are free of side effects and have been used in healing for centuries.

Pharmaceutical drugs are based upon the same biochemical research that alternative medicine uses. But, drug companies can't profit from natural substances, so they create synthetic molecules, which distort brain chemistry.

Alternative, or natural healing, is the wave of the future. What seems unusual and different now may well become the standard of care in the future. Why wait when so much is already available today?

"Dr. Suka" Chapel-Horst
December 2013

Etowah, North Carolina

TRICK or TREAT

What your doctor isn't telling you about mood-altering medications.

Is your doctor treating you or tricking you? Let's begin with a few facts.

In the 1952 edition of the **Diagnostic and Statistical Manual**, the psychiatrist's "bible", 106 mental disorders were listed. In the 2013 fifth edition, 297 mental disorders are listed, an increase of 191 mental disorders.

As more and more medications are developed for mental illness, more mental diagnoses are "generated" to permit physicians to legally prescribe these medications.

So, human traits that were once considered normal have now been given mental illness labels. It used to be that a shy or introverted person was simply shy and introverted. Now shyness and introversion is a mental illness... (for which there is a medication).

"At [this] rate, almost 50 percent of Americans (46.4% to be exact) will have a diagnosable mental illness in their lifetimes,..." states Robin S. Rosenberg PhD. ABPP, Clinical Psychologist.

The rate of diagnosing children and teens who are bipolar is now 40 times greater than it was in 2001, despite the debate over whether the disorder even exists in children.

As Slate's Christopher Lane wrote in a critique of the DSM-V, "If you spend hours online, have sex more frequently than aging psychiatrists, and moan incessantly that the federal government can't account for all its TARP funds, take heed: you may soon be classed among the 48 million Americans the APA (American Psychiatric Association) already considers mentally ill."

The National Institute of Mental Health argues that the DSM represents an unscientific and subjective system, but permits the sale of more prescription drugs.

Mayo Clinic research shows that 70% of Americans are taking one prescription drug, 50% of Americans are taking two prescription drugs, and 20% of Americans are taking five prescription drugs. (CBS News 6/20/2013)

The number one medications people are taking are antidepressants, pain-killing opioids, and antibiotics. In 2012 there were more opiate addicted than alcohol addicted people in treatment. Note that antidepressants, benzodiazepines and opioids are addictive after approximately just thirty days.

As all these mood altering drugs became available, the promise we heard from the pharmaceutical companies and our physicians was that *"wonder drugs will make us well"*.

In fact, as the number of mood and mind altering pharmaceutical medications have increased, so have mental and emotional disorders increased. I have to ask, who stands to gain from increased emotional and mental disorders?

Some readers want proof of what I'm writing about, and so, at this point I want to refer you to a definitive book on the subject. *Anatomy of an Epidemic* - Magic Bullets, Psychiatric Drugs, and The Astonishing Rise of Mental Illness in America by Robert Whitaker published in 2010.

Another excellent resource is *Overdosed America, The Broken Promise of American Medicine* by John Abramson, MD.

Research shows us that rather than *fixing* chemical imbalances in the brain, the drugs *create* imbalances. In addition, the studies show that "pills" *worsen* long-term outcomes, at least in the aggregate.

What does this mean? It means that in the beginning, there may be symptom relief, but, long term use of "pills" creates a dependence from which the brain cannot recover.

So, what's happening in the brain? There are over 100 billion neurons in the brain. Neurons, or brain cells, are not connected to each other. Neurotransmitters, of which there are over a hundred, are the brain's messengers. They are the chemicals that carry messages from one neuron to another. These neurotransmitters are made of proteins and proteins are made up of amino acids, the same proteins and amino acids that are found in our food.

Some of the emotional and mental symptoms that are due to brain chemistry imbalances of these neurotransmitters are:

- Depression
- Craving
- Insomnia
- Anxiety
- Low energy
- Unmotivated
- Lack of concentration
- Poor memory
- Hyperactivity
- Irritability

- Negative thinking
- Hopelessness
- Panic attacks
- Paranoia
- Obsessiveness
- Compulsiveness
- Hallucinations
- Anger outbursts
- Violence
- Suicidal thinking

FOUR NEUROTRANSMITTERS

Let's take a look at just four of the major neurotransmitters. **Dopamine, Serotonin, GABA,** and the **Endorphins.**

Dopamine is the "Energizer Bunny" neurotransmitter. It's a "feel good" chemical that stimulates, excites and motivates us. It helps us to concentrate and take action. **Dopamine is the brain's natural cocaine.**

Symptoms of a dopamine DEFICIENCY are:
- Reduced ability to feel pleasure
- Flat, bored, apathetic and low enthusiasm
- Depressed
- Low drive and motivation
- Procrastination
- Difficulty concentrating
- Slowed thinking
- Poor memory
- Low energy
- Unmotivated
- Shy/introverted
- Low libido or impotence
- Sleep too much

- Trouble getting out of bed
- Put on weight easily
- Mentally and physically easily fatigued
- Family history of alcoholism/ADD/ADHD

Dopamine deficiency SOLUTIONS people use are:
- Sugars
- Caffeine
- Sodas
- Refined carbohydrates (doughnuts, French fries, chips, etc.)
- Shopping
- Gambling
- Antidepressants
- Amphetamines
- Ritalin, Adderall, Concerta, etc.
- Marijuana
- Tobacco
- Alcohol

Serotonin is the brain's "Sunshine" neurotransmitter. It relaxes us, affects our moods, sleep, appetite, and our perception. **Serotonin is the brain's natural antidepressant.**

Symptoms of a serotonin DEFICIENCY are:
- Depression
- Anxiety
- Irritability
- Impatience
- Impulsiveness
- Inability to concentrate
- Weight gain or unexplained weight loss
- Overeating and/or carbohydrate cravings
- Poor dream recall
- Insomnia

Serotonin deficiency SOLUTIONS people use are:
- Overeating
- Sugar
- Refined Carbs
- Marijuana
- Tobacco
- Alcohol
- Antidepressants: such as Paxil, Zoloft, Prozac, Wellbutrin, etc.

GABA is the brain's "Chill Out" neurotransmitter. It's a sedative and it reduces anxiety. **GABA is the brain's natural Valium.**

Symptoms of a GABA DEFICIENCY are:
- Anxiety or panic
- Difficulty relaxing
- Easily stressed or overwhelmed
- Overworked or pressured
- Body uptight or stiff
- Sometimes feel weak or shaky
- Increased stress if skip a meal
- Bothered by loud noises, lights, too much activity

GABA Deficiency SOLUTIONS people use are:
- Sugar
- Sodas
- Refined Carbs
- Benzos (Sedative Hypnotics) Valium, Ativan, Xanax, Klonipin, Restoril, etc.
- Neurontin
- Barbiturates: Fioricet for migraines
- Soma (relaxes the brain not muscles)
- Sleep Aids: Ambien, Lunesta, or Prosom, etc.
- Marijuana
- Tobacco   Alcohol

Endorphins are the "Love Bug" neurotransmitters. They provide comfort and pleasure. They are the **brain's natural pain killers (opiates)** for both emotional and physical pain.

Symptoms of an endorphin DEFICIENCY are:
- Discomfort
- Persistent pain – emotional and physical
- Stress and frustration
- Low interest, focus, concentration

Endorphin Deficiency SOLUTIONS people use are:
- Sugar
- Sodas
- Refined Carbohydrates
- Opiates – Heroin, Oxycontin, Percocet, etc.
- Marijuana
- Tobacco
- Alcohol

SOME MORE FACTS

The U.S. is the most medicated nation in the world even though symptom relief is often short term, the side effects require more medications, and medications don't restore brain chemistry. In fact, they further *distort* brain chemistry.

People on mind and mood altering medications frequently complain of brain fog, or of being drowsy or groggy. They have poor memory, and difficulty with focus and concentration. They often have low motivation and low energy as a result of taking these medications.

According to the Physician's Desk Reference some antidepressant side-effects are:

- Depression
- Suicide
- Hostility
- Hallucinations
- Paranoid reactions
- Personality disorder
- Psychosis
- Delusions
- Confusion agitation
- Sleep disorder
- Ataxia
- Apathy
- Neuralgia
- Abnormal EEG
- Coma
- Dystonia
- Stupor

Think of watching an advertisement for a medication on TV. All the time you are focused on the pretty pictures of people having a lovely, relaxing time picnicking at the lake, the following is being spoken in a soft and soothing voice.

SIDE EFFECTS of SEROQUEL

Elderly patients with dementia-related psychosis-increased risk of death, depression, suicidal thoughts or actions, unusual changes in behavior, agitation, and irritability, sudden changes in mood, behaviors, thoughts, or feelings, stroke in elderly people with dementia, high fever; excessive sweating, stiff muscles; confusion; changes in pulse, heart rate, and blood pressure, high blood sugar and diabetes, increases in triglycerides and in LDL (bad) cholesterol and decreases in HDL (good) cholesterol, weight gain, movements you cannot control in your face, tongue, or other body parts, feeling dizzy or lightheaded upon standing, decreases in white blood cells (which can be fatal), or trouble swallowing, drowsiness, dry mouth, constipation, dizziness, increased appetite, upset stomach, fatigue, disturbance in speech and language, and stuffy nose.

This is not a complete summary of safety information. **So, call your doctor for a prescription, now.**

If you were to listen to a car dealer on TV giving this advertisement, what would you do?

This car has no gas in the gas tank, no air in the tires, no oil in the crankcase, no water in the radiator. Rusted throughout. Batteries are dead. Needs new engine, transmission, brakes, hoses, belts. Seat upholstery is dirty and worn through. Windows are cracked. Lights don't work. Trunk doesn't latch. Fender is falling off. Needs new wiper blades. Smells of cigarette smoke. Doesn't start. There's a hole in the floorboards. **Call your auto dealer and purchase this car today.**

Let's take a look at the adverse effects from prescription medications. They are the fourth leading cause of hospital deaths topped   only by heart disease, cancer and stroke. The death rate from prescription drugs, taken as directed, was three times greater than from all illicit drugs combined. (2008, Florida Medical Examiners Commission, Federal: Agency for Healthcare Research & Quality, The National Academy of Sciences' Institute of Medicine)

What do these mood and mind altering substances have in common? Antidepressants, benzodiazepines, antipsychotics, alcohol, cocaine, and heroin. They are all drugs! Legal and illegal; all are the same.

What else do these substances have in common? They are addictive and have withdrawal symptoms.   They manipulate brain chemistry, destroy brain cells, and *make the condition chronic over time.*

An examination of the mass shootings that have occurred in the past 15 years shows that every shooter was being medicated and had had a recent increase or decrease in a psychiatric medication.

Since the advent of SSRI antidepressants, there is an 840% increase in the rate of violence among those taking these drugs. That includes violence toward others as well as violent suicide. (Depressed individuals, who are not on SSRI medications, while they may commit suicide, do not commit *violent* suicide.)

In the U.S. we have a war on drugs, a Drug Enforcement Administration, and a Federal Drug Administration. Drugs are getting the government's attention, yet physicians are allowed to legally prescribe mood altering drugs!! What's the difference between approved and illegal drugs?

HOW DO MOOD-ALTERING DRUGS WORK?

Let's take a look at how some specific medications for depression act upon specific neurotransmitters.

All neurons, or brain cells, both send and receive neurotransmitters (NT). In the natural state one brain cell sends the NT to the next brain cell and that cell repeats the process for all the cells that handle that particular NT. What isn't taken up by the receiving NT is reabsorbed back into the sending brain cell. Nothing is left in the space between the cells.

Let's consider how some SSRI's (Selective Serotonin Reuptake Inhibiter) medications such as Celexa, Lexapro, Prozac, Luvox, Paxil, and Zoloft, to name a few, work.

After the sending neuron (brain cell) releases Serotonin into the space between cells, called a synapse, SSRI medications block the sending cell's "doorway" so that the serotonin can't return back into it. This leaves serotonin in the space between cells.

The receiving cell accepts and absorbs what it can leaving the excess "hanging out" in the synapse. The idea is that the receiving cell will have more serotonin available to absorb. In other words, the SSRI keeps more serotonin available at the receiving cell's door so that the person can get a bigger lift from depression.

However, by holding the unabsorbed serotonin in the synaptic space, some of the serotonin escapes into other parts of the brain and is lost. Some of the serotonin left in the synapse becomes degraded. This, then, creates a *loss* of serotonin.

The result is that the serotonin level is decreased over time. Therefore, the SSRI dosage has to be increased to get the same effect or one has to switch to a more powerful medication.

So let's look at some other antidepressants. Cymbalta, Effexor, Wellbutrin, and Remeron, to name a few, have the same effect on the neurotransmitter dopamine. They block the reabsorption of dopamine into the sending neuron.

The result is that the dopamine level is decreased over time. Therefore, the antidepressant dosage has to be increased to get the same effect or one has to switch to a more powerful medication.

Alcohol stimulates the secretion of dopamine. To protect from an overproduction of dopamine, the brain will decrease its own production over time. The receiving brain cell also closes some doors so that less and less can be absorbed. Then alcohol consumption has to be increased to get the same effect or one has to switch to a more powerful form of alcohol. (See the book *How to Quit Drinking for Good and Feel Good* listed in the Resources section of this book.)

Antidepressants, benzodiazepines, opiates, and antipsychotics manipulate brain chemistry but they do not restore neurotransmitter levels to normal.

Alcohol, cocaine, methamphetamine, benzodiazepines, and heroin manipulate brain chemistry but they do not restore neurotransmitter levels to normal.

The brain is always seeking to adapt. It's called homeostasis. However, over time, the brain is so manipulated by drugs, legal and illegal, that it can't return to a normal state on its own.

This leaves a person in a chronic state of depression, whether it's caused by emotional and mental disorders, or alcoholism and drug abuse.

Mood altering drugs may be useful for short-term symptom relief but the goal should be to return brain chemistry to normal, thus eliminating the need for drugs.

Women on antidepressants have a 45% increased chance of stroke and the risk of dying is in increased by 32%. (AMA)

GETTING OFF ANTIDEPRESSANTS

All antidepressants are addictive after about thirty days. That's the CATCH-22. When a person tries to stop taking their antidepressants, withdrawal symptoms will occur. The timing of the symptoms depends upon the half-life of the drug.

If the symptoms are moderate to severe, people, and the physician, think that the depressive symptoms have returned. Not true. It takes four to six weeks for the underlying depressive symptoms to reoccur. What are being experienced are *withdrawal symptoms.*

Most physicians will encourage their patients to get back on their medicine, and even increase the dosage. Physicians are informed by pharmaceutical reps who have no medical or biochemical training at all. They are parrots for the drug companies who don't want patients going off their medications. There is rarely any training on how to wean patients off medications.

I recommend an excellent book, written by a Harvard medical physician, to inform and help people get off their antidepressants. It has everything one needs to know and more than most physicians know.

Please don't attempt to quit your antidepressants without reading this book first. The book is *The Antidepressant Solution* by Dr. Joseph Glenmullen, MD and it's available at www.alibris.com/

Before statin drugs, the healthy cholesterol level was 130. As statin drugs were developed the pharmaceutical companies arranged with the

AMA (American Medical Association) to lover the "healthy" cholesterol level to 100 so that statin drugs could be legally prescribed. We now know that Statin drugs increase:

- Hormonal imbalances
- Stroke
- Suicide
- Violent behavior
- Parkinson's Disease

So, *EAT EGGS!!* They're healthy.

The problem is not the medications; the problem is physicians:
- Failure to find cause by investigation/testing
- Lack of education
- Misdiagnosing
- Wrong medication
- Over-prescribing
- Failure to oversee
- Disinclination to stop medication
- Ignorance

And, the problem is pharmaceutical:
- Failure to disclose true trial results
- Marketing strategy
- Government lobbying
- Greed

Paul McHugh, a professor and former Psychiatrist in Chief at Johns Hopkins Hospital, says the DSM-5 fails to distinguish between the underlying causes of the symptoms associated with its diagnoses.

SO, WHAT'S THE SOLUTION?

The solution is to rebuild imbalanced brain chemistry. We have to restore neurotransmitter and hormone levels to normal, naturally. But how?

Using antidepressant and antipsychotic drugs without determining the underlying cause is like painting over the rust on a car.

SOME SUGGESTED LABORATORY TESTING includes:

- **DHEA and Cortisol Level**

Cortisol is the major stress hormone that wreaks havoc on the brain when stress is chronic. DHEA is a hormone that manages the cortisol level. However, DHEA reaches its peak of production when we are in our 20's and then decreases as we age. Once testing is done to determine one's DHEA level, a supplement can be taken to raise DHEA to the level we once had in our 20's.

An all-natural food supplement for managing one's cortisol level is listed in the Resources portion of this book.

Chronic stress and high cortisol levels are responsible for up to 95% of all illness, disease, mental misery, and premature aging. For more information watch the DVD and read the book called *The Gift – A Sound Mind for Life* which is listed in the Resources portion of this book.

- **Thyroid: TSH, Free T3, Free T4**

If the thyroid gland isn't working properly, nothing else will work either. The most informative test is TSH, along with a Free T3 and Free T4 level. This is a laboratory test. See Resources.

- **Neurotransmitter Levels**

For more information read the book *"Why Do I Feel This Way?"* – *Natural Relief from Moods and Depression* which includes a Mood Meter for testing neurotransmitter levels. (See Resources) One can also get laboratory testing for these levels.

Nutrient Evaluation

A nutrient evaluation can assist in the development of micronutrient and nutritional protocols. This is a laboratory test. See Resources.

- **Hormone Levels**

Hormone levels should be checked, especially with females, it they are having difficult menses, or menopause symptoms.

- **Toxic Metals**

We all carry toxins in our bodies due to mercury in our teeth, foods, environmental chemicals, fluoride in the water, and much more. A hair analysis or blood test will be helpful. See Resources.

Individuals with **bipolar depression, schizophrenia, autism, Asperger's** and **severe depressio**n should have the following tests performed.
- Copper/Zinc Levels
- Histamine Level (Complete Metabolic Screening)
- Pyroluria (Vitamin B's and Zinc loss through urine)

If diagnosed with **Pyroluria**, the condition can be corrected very quickly and naturally with complete relief from all pyroluria caused symptoms. For more information on histimines and Pyroluria see the self-help manual *"Why Do I Feel This Way?" – Natural Healing for Optimal Health and Relief from Moods and Depression* listed in Resources.

All **Schizophrenics** are gluten sensitive. When gluten is removed from the diet some people diagnosed with this disorder become completely symptom free.

Port-partum depression is commonly due to a copper/zinc imbalance. A high copper level is normal during pregnancy. When the copper level fails to return to normal after the birth of the baby, the mother will experience post-partum depression which, if improperly treated, can last for months. Most doctors treat it with an anti-depressant.

23

However, the depression can usually be relieved within one to three weeks by simply rebalancing the copper/zinc level with all natural food supplements. Consult an integrative or functional medicine provider for instructions.

(See the Resources section of this book for information on **Bi-Polar Depression** and an all-natural food supplementation program that is helping thousands recover from this severe disorder. Also see the DVD *DEPRESSION CURE* to discover ten different types of depression and ten different types of cure.)

More information about these and other tests is available in the manual *"Why Do I Feel This Way?" – Natural Healing for Optimal Health and Relief from Moods and Depression.* (See Resources at the end of this book.) The manual includes ten written self-tests to assist in determining what some underlying causes might be.

Solutions for many of the tests are given in the manual and if people test positive to a few of the tests, they will be directed to their healthcare practitioner for further testing. Taking the manual and test results to one's physician may be very helpful. The tests include:
- Carb Addiction
- Candida
- Allergies
- Hypoglycemia
- Hypothyroid
- Alcohol Screening
- Pyroluria
- High Histamine
- Low Histamine
- Adrenal Insufficiency

HYPOGLYCEMIA

Hypoglycemia, or low blood sugar, occurs when we eat lots of sugar, in any form, on a regular basis. Too much insulin is released to metabolize the sugar. When all the sugar is metabolized, the result is excess insulin and low blood sugar. That's the condition called hypoglycemia. Note that there can be serious repercussions from low blood sugar.

Symptoms of low blood sugar are:
- Unprovoked anxieties
- Exhaustion
- Mental confusion
- Forgetfulness
- Irritability
- Insomnia
- Constant worrying
- Internal trembling
- DEPRESSION
- ANGRY OUTBURSTS
- VIOLENCE
- SUICIDE

You and your mind are precious. Protect them with knowledge and good choices.

PRIMARY BRAIN REPAIR

We need to rebalance brain chemistry with nature's building blocks. *"Babies are not made from Prozac."*

We begin with the magic of aminos. You'll recall that all proteins are made of amino acids. Amino acids, and only amino acids, are nature's building blocks for neurotransmitters. Become an amino acid addict (AAA). Rebuild your neurotransmitters the only way possible, by doing it naturally. For example, look at how the following amino acids lead to the creation of our four neurotransmitters.

The amino acid **L-Tyrosine** leads to the formation of the neurotransmitter **Dopamine**.

The amino acid **L-Tryptophan** leads to the formation of the neurotransmitter **Serotonin**.

The amino acid **GABA** leads to the formation of the neurotransmitter **GABA**.

The amino acid **Phenylalanine** leads to the formation of the **Endorphins**.

To aid in restoring brain chemistry with amino acids, the book *"Why Do I Feel This Way?" – Natural Healing for Optimal Health and Relief from Moods and Depression* contains a Mood Meter with written tests to help you discover what neurotransmitters you may be low in, if any. The written tests are very accurate because they are based on the specific symptoms that are caused by specific neurotransmitter deficiencies.

The book also contains amino acid protocols - the what, when, and how to use amino acids. Please be aware that people should not just go out and buy amino acids. While they have no side effects when taken **appropriately**, some amino acids should **not** be taken under certain conditions or if a person is on some specific medications. If a person doesn't need an amino acid and takes it, she may have a short-term (minutes) negative reaction. That's why the book also contains a complete "**precautions**" list to check out before taking the aminos. This book is truly a self-help, how-to manual, easy to read and understand.

When buying amino acids and supplements, always choose quality over cost. Most cheap aminos are made in China. They're cheap because they have:

- No quality control
- No supervision
- No oversight
- No or little amino acids in the capsules
- No or little herbs in the capsules

THREE TIPS

To give you an opportunity to see just how potent natural substances can be, here are three tips to get you started.

Do you have the blues, blahs, or <u>mild</u> depression?
Take Vitamin D3 15,000 – 20,000 IU daily
When recovered take 5000 IU daily for maintenance, or more as needed.

Do you have cravings for sugar, sweets, or alcohol?
Take the amino acid L-GLUTAMINE, 500 mg powder, or more, under the tongue, as needed, to prevent or eliminate cravings. Open up a capsule and place the powder under your tongue. (Do not take if bipolar or have lymphatic cancer.)

Do you have anxiety or panic attacks?
Take Inositol Powder (Vitamin B) 1000 mg under your tongue, up to four times daily, or as needed, and L-Glutamine powder, 500 to 1500 mg, under the tongue, as needed. Open up a capsule and place the powder under your tongue. (Do not take L-Glutamine if you are bipolar.)

As with any substance, immediately stop it if you have any negative reactions, a rare, quickly relieved, occurrence.

NEURONUTRIENTS

Amino acids can't work alone. In order for them to be metabolized, co-factors – the vitamins, minerals, enzymes, essential fatty acids, and trace elements - are required.

For example, let's look at just the Vitamins B. When there is a deficiency in these nutrients, multiple symptoms may develop such as:

Emotional Symptoms of a Vitamin B Deficiency
- Confusion
- Poor concentration

- Poor memory
- Depression
- Insomnia
- Anxiety
- Agitation
- Impulsive
- Anger
- Irritability
- Quarrelsome
- Mood swings
- Panic attacks
- Obsessive-compulsive

Physical Symptoms of a Vitamin B Deficiency

- Hyperactivity
- Headache
- Fatigue
- Insomnia
- Convulsions
- Agitation
- Decreased sex drive
- Tension
- Dizziness
- Gastric ulcers
- High blood pressure
- High cholesterol
- Arteriosclerosis
- Constipation
- Hair loss
- Skin eruptions
- Kidney /Liver impairment
- Extreme nervous exhaustion

Sugar is the #1 Medication and #1 Killer

Sugar is four times more addictive than cocaine. It's a POISON leading to:

- Obesity
- Diabetes
- Cancer
- Alzheimer's
- DEPRESSION
- RAGE
- VIOLENCE

Our physician told us that if all his patients would cut down or quit their sugar intake, he would lose 70% of his patients. He's right. Before even considering taking any mind or mood altering medications, stop eating sugar and sugar products. Your symptoms may decrease altogether.

The Standard American Diet (SAD) is junk food. Americans have the poorest nutritional standard in the world and the most malnutrition. For too many families, fast foods and junk foods are the family's only meals. We see the results in the increase of childhood disorders, obesity (obese people are malnourished), heart problems, diabetes, cancer, and ultimately in dementia and Alzheimer's. Learning problems, behavioral problems, and violence have increased with the over-consumption of these non-foods.

Eat three wholesome meals daily, not one or two. The most important meal is breakfast and all meals should contain protein and healthy fats, such as real butter, chicken fat, and cheese, for example (if not allergic to dairy).

Allergies, alone, can be responsible for almost all symptoms. Allergies to wheat and dairy are the most common. The manual mentioned above includes both a written test and instructions for food elimination tests for allergies. Simple, costing nothing, these tests may lead to the resolution of many symptoms and disorders.

Water

Drink six to eight glasses of water every day. Our bodies are about 70% water. When the level is too low we can experience stress related symptoms.

"Let your medicine be your food. Let your food be your medicine."
Hippocrates

Homeopathic and naturopathic remedies are natural and holistic products that can assist in recovery. Contact a qualified practitioner for assistance. Don't attempt to be your own doctor. Avoid a "little dab of this and a little dab of that". We are holistic in nature. Knowing how to put all the pieces together, like a picture puzzle, requires knowledge of the picture we want to create.

BODY WORK

Exercise or walking is a major part of recovery. However, I know that many people don't like to exercise. For those who do, fine. For those who don't, forty minutes of brisk walking four days a week will do it. Walk fast enough to keep the heart rate up. Breaking a little sweat is a good sign that you're getting a decent workout.

STRESS RELIEF

Recovery is all about stress management. Take advantage of some of these suggestions:

- Yoga
- Tai Chi
- Qigong
- Meditation
- Breathing exercises
- Spiritual rejuvenation

- EMDR
- Reiki
- Massage
- Reflexology
- Chiropractic
- Acupuncture
- Quantum Touch
- Polarity Therapy
- Therapeutic Touch
- Cranial Sacral Therapy
- Meridian tapping www.eft.mercola.com
- Myofascial Trigger Point Therapy
- Infra-Red Dry-Heat Saunas

INTEGRATIVE MEMORY THERAPY®

Present day physical, emotional, and mental pain and suffering are the result of unresolved issues from our past. It can be called Post Traumatic Stress. That "past" can be yesterday, or years ago. The unresolved issues may have occurred during our early formative years or in the womb.

Yes, we recorded the feelings, thoughts, and words mother experienced during the time we were a tiny fetus in her womb. We simply recorded these, and all that we saw, heard, and felt during the first seven years of our life. These experiences became our history and our truths because we didn't yet have a conscious mind to discriminate. The stories created beliefs about ourselves and our ability to live in the world, even though the beliefs may have been wrong or harmful.

Sometimes these memories or "stories" may appear to be past life trauma stories that are seeking resolution. It makes no difference whether the stories are fantasy or real. If the stories coming from our own unconscious mind are left unresolved, they create unhealthy survival patterns and suffering in our present lives. These unhealthy survival patterns can show up as addictions, cancer, arthritis, anorexia, depression, PTSD, AD(H)D, for example. In fact, every illness and every disorder is the result of unresolved prior trauma.

Integrative Memory Therapy® gets to the originating source of present day issues, allowing for healing and transformation. Unlike other medical and alternative modalities, this process resolves the root of the problem. Healing in the present takes place because the underlying cause is no longer present.

Integrative Memory Therapy® is not regression, nor is it hypnosis. Clients are fully conscious at all times. The therapist guides clients to resolve their own source traumas. The result is a transformed life in the present. This therapy must be conducted in person. It cannot be conducted via Skype or telephone.

For more information contact Dr. Suka at 417-890-3254 or go to www.IMRIWellness.org. Additional information and testimonials are available on the web site.

SUMMARY
All mood and mind altering drugs are drugs, whether legal or illegal. All drugs have side effects, are addictive, and lead to chronic conditions over time. They all distort brain chemistry and none of them restore brain chemistry back to normal.

The only way to relieve unwanted symptoms and restore brain chemistry to normal is by using specific formulas consisting of amino acids, vitamins, minerals, fatty acids, enzymes, and trace elements, plus healthy nutrition, exercise, and stress relief.

Please share this information with others and help to enhance someone's life. It's never too late. *Dr. Suka*

December 2013
Etowah, North Carolina

RESOURCES

LABORATORY TESTING

SOME RECOMMENDED TESTS
- DHEA and Cortisol Levels
- Thyroid: TSH, Free T3, Free T4
- Neurotransmitter Levels
- Nutrient Evaluation
- Hormone Levels
- Toxic Metals (Hair and blood analysis)
- Histimine, Pyroluria, and Copper/Zinc levels

SUGGESTED LABORTORIES

Direct Health: www.pyroluriatesting.com
Tests can be ordered directly by the individual on line, through a healthcare provider, or through Dr. Suka. Insurance may cover these tests.

Sanesco Health: www.sanescohealth.com
Sanesco Health offers testing for neurotransmitters and adrenal insufficiency (DHEA and Cortisol). Tests can be ordered through a healthcare provider or through Dr. Suka. Insurance coverage is available.

NeuroScience: www.neurorelief.com
NeuroScience offers neurotransmitter testing. Tests can be ordered through a healthcare provider. Insurance coverage may be available.

Genova Diagnostics: www.gdx.net
Tests can be ordered through a healthcare provider. Insurance coverage may be available.

Life Extension: www.lef.org
Life Extension offers a large variety of tests available to the public without a prescription.

Vitamin D Council: www.vitamindcouncil.com
Inexpensive and accurate Vitamin D testing. No prescription necessary.

TO ORDER HIGH QUALITY SUPPLEMENTS LISTED IN THIS BOOK, CALL ANOVA HEALTH AT 864-408-8320.

Food supplements listed in all of our books can be purchased through Anova Health, also providing WHOLE FOOD supplements. Request a catalog.

Simply call Anova Health and give them the CODE. **Drsuka5** Your order will be shipped the same day, no delays. You will automatically receive a **5% discount and free shipping,** saving you the extra cost of buying supplements of the very best quality. To get these benefits, you must call in your order.

All supplements are of the highest quality available and are suitable for vegetarians. They are free of wheat gluten, soy, milk/dairy, corn, sodium, sugar, starch, artificial coloring, preservatives, and flavoring. I highly recommend the following supplements available through Anova Health.

Amino Acids: All of the amino acids that are listed in my two "how-to" manuals and other books can be ordered through Anova Health. Of course, they can be purchased in many other places, but for the highest quality and purest products, I recommend Anova Health. You may pay a little more, but you will use less and get better results with high quality products.

AvinoCort for managing elevated Cortisol levels caused by chronic stress. Lowering one's cortisol level slows down the aging process and helps to prevent dementia and Alzheimer's. Why use this product? This is a very advanced, stem cell product. Ask the folks at Anova Health for more information if you like. I highly recommend this product for reducing the effects of chronic stress.

Inositol Powder is a normal vitamin B. It is a precursor to GABA, the brain's natural Valium. If you have anxiety, worries, even panic attacks, your inositol level is probably too low. Taking 1000 mg up to four times daily can improve relaxation and reduce anxiety, naturally.

High Potency Hemp Oil with Cannabidiol (CBD): Legal everywhere and has no measurable THC or psycho-active effects. Cannabidiol relieves or cures over 100 symptoms and disorders. Comes as oil and capsules. An excellent balm is also available for topical use. To learn more about the advantages of hemp oil with Cannabidiol versus marijuana with TCH for medicinal support, order the Bottom Line Book *Cannabinoids – The Hundredth Monkey Cure* (see page 54) available on our web site. This product, combined with vitamin D3, may be the closest there is to "magic medicine". Recommended for drug and alcohol detoxing and recovery, as well.

CaliQuil - California Poppy 500 mg Capsules Restores Rest. Prevails over pain. Traditional analgesic and sleep aid. This amazing product really works. Take it before bedtime and see the results. (Does not produce opium, physical dependence, or addiction.)

Acute Pain Relief, a King Bio homeopathic cream, gives excellent relief from joint pain.

Call 864-408-8320 to order these and other products from Anova Health. (If you order on-line, you won't get the discount or free shipping.)

Use the code **drsuka5** to order.

OTHER SUGGESTED RESOURCES FOR QUALITY SUPPLEMENTS
Call and request free catalogs. Order by telephone or on-line.

- Life Extension: www.lef.org 1-800-678-8989
- Bronson Vitamins: www.bronsonvitamins.com 1-800-235-3200
- Cayenne Company: www.cayennecompany.com
  1-800-229-3663
- For Highest Quality Amino Acids Call: Dr. Suka at 417-380-3254 or 417-894-8501
- True Hope: www.TrueHope.com for **Bi-Polar disorder**

ALCOHOL RECOVERY PROGRAMS

***ARISE* Alcohol Recovery** offers two Do-It-Yourself, at home, recovery programs. These include both a Self-Managed Program and a Managed Program.

***ARISE* Alcohol Recovery** also offers an Out-patient Program for individuals who have been through one or more treatment programs, or have made good attempts at recovery through AA, and have relapsed. The program can also serve as an aftercare program for someone coming out of treatment but who is not yet ready to return home.

All programs are based on biochemical restoration of the brain using micronutrient and nutrition therapy, body work, whole life skills, and Integrative Memory Therapy®.

For more information and testimonials, go to:
www.AriseAlcoholRecovery.com

DVD
Depression Cure
Ten Different Sources / Ten Different Approaches   Get Real Results
Your Guide to Finding and Treating the Real Underlying Cause
PowerPoint Presentation by Suka Chapel-Horst, RN, PhD, QMHP, CPLT

Don't waste time using the wrong approach to recovery. "Dr. Suka" pinpoints the different underlying sources of depression which must be treated uniquely and appropriately in order to fully recover without the use of pharmaceuticals. These inter-related causes require different treatment approaches to achieve permanent cure. Don't waste precious time, money, and hopes. Get to the root source from the start and find out how to recover naturally. DVD comes with a resource list.

BOOK (234 pages)
Take a Leap of Faith
Wellness Simplified
by Suka Chapel-Horst, RN, PhD, QMHP, CPLT

If your emotional, mental, or physical health isn't what you wish it to be, you'll find practical suggestions for regaining or maintaining optimal health in this remarkable book. The topics include:

- Halt Premature Aging Now
- Want More Sunshine in Your Life?
- The Cookie Monster - Hypoglycemia
- Five Simple Steps to Optimal Health
- Enjoy Life More
- Your Body Type: Seven Dwarfs and Superman
- Fear versus Love
- Relief from Depression
- Stretching to Wellness
- Bodyguards Got You Covered?
- Bodyguard Banquet
- What are you Hoarding in your Mental House?
- Prevent Dementia and Alzheimer's
- The Hundredth Monkey Cure – Cannabinoids
- Is There a Cure for Alcoholism?
- Color – The Hidden Persuader
- The Ultimate Healing – Integrative Memory and Past Lives Therapy®
- Take a Leap of Faith
- What I know for Sure
- …and more

In the most delightful and warm way, Dr. Suka "talks" about the topics closest to our minds and hearts.   This book includes transcripts from 24 of her recent Unity.FM international radio shows. You won't want to put this book down.

BOOKS

"Why Do I Feel This Way?" - Natural Relief from Moods and Depression by Suka Chapel-Horst, RN, PhD, QMHP

Moods, cravings, chronic depression, aches, pains and other symptoms are caused by treatable and reversible deficiencies in brain chemistry.

If your brain is low in "feel good" chemicals, you may experience moodiness, sadness, anxiety, overeating, insomnia, irritability, anger, lack of focus and concentration, poor memory, loneliness, decreased sex drive, lack of motivation, racing thoughts, suicidal thoughts, and more.

Find out which "feel good" brain chemicals you may be deficient in. Experience the power of amino acids to restore brain chemistry without medications. Discover the foods and basic food supplements that can restore your life to normal. The guidelines are clear, easy to understand and follow. This book may be all you need to achieve optimal health.

Avoid medication side effects, serious dangers, and addictive qualities. The only way to restore optimal health is by deleting poisonous nonfoods and feeding the brain the natural substances it needs to function normally.

The book includes:
- Ten Written Tests to Uncover the Underlying Cause
- Neurotransmitter Testing
- Amino Acid Formulas
- Nutritional Co-Factor Formulas
- Three Nutritional Programs
- Allergy and Candida Repair
- Seventeen Fun and Effective Stress-Reducing Exercises

This book can be ordered through:
www.IMRIWellness.org
www.AriseAlcoholRecovery.com

BOOKS
How to Quit Drinking for Good and Feel Good
By Suka Chapel-Horst, RN, PhD, QMHP

Live at Home

Keep it Private

Continue Normal Activities

Make it Affordable

Much of what we thought we knew about alcoholism and substance abuse is now obsolete. Neuroscience and biochemistry have found the underlying cause of all addictions and thirty-plus years of experience have given us the recovery method that is getting up to 85% recovery rates.

Shame, blame, and guilt be gone. Anger and hurt can change to healing, compassion and forgiveness when the real cause of addictions is understood. Addictions are not caused by a mental illness, nor are they caused by a lack of will power, a character defect, or a moral weakness.

Sobriety is not recovery. "One day at a time" struggling, white knuckling, dry drunk behaviors, depression, insomnia, anxiety, cravings, and other symptoms lead to relapse. With the new understanding of addictions, these, and other symptoms can be relieved and prevented, naturally, without the side effects and addictive qualities of prescription medications.

This book contains ten written tests to determine one's underlying biochemical imbalances and a step-by-step guide for gaining and maintaining lasting recovery without the symptoms that lead to relapse. Normal brain chemistry is restored with the natural building blocks of micronutrients and healthy nutrition. This program uses the most successful method of recovery available anywhere. Motivated and determined individuals can recover once and for all.

Written tests included in this book are:
- Alcohol Screening
- Carbohydrate Addiction
- Hypoglycemia
- Hypothyroid
- Candida
- Allergies
- Pyroluria
- High Histamine
- Low Histamine
- Attention Deficit (Hyperactivity) Disorder

This book can be ordered through:
www.IMRIWellness.org
www.AriseAlcoholRecovery.com

BOTTOM LINE BOOKS

BOOK/DVD
Wellness Simplified
How Food affects Moods, Bodies and Behaviors
PowerPoint Presentation by Suka Chapel-Horst, RN, PhD, QMHP, CPLT

Think what you eat doesn't matter? Fast food, junk food, sodas, and pizza are the voices of violence, crime, and suicide, as well as obesity, joint pain, insomnia, anxiety, diabetes, depression, cancer, and *you name it!*

What we eat affects the quality of our lives. Sick and tired of feeling sick and tired? Are children's behaviors getting out of hand? Are school grades going down? It's OK. There's a solution and it's not rocket science.

This little book can change lives for the better, right now. The solution makes sense and it's doable. Say "goodbye" to moods, sickness, and unwanted behaviors. Say "hello" to good health and happiness.

BOOK
Say Goodbye to Moods and Depression
by Suka Chapel-Horst, RN, PhD, QMHP, CPLT

The only way to restore optimal health is by deleting poisonous nonfoods and feeding the brain the natural substances from which it is made.

Babies are made from food, not Prozac. After birth, why do we switch from the natural building blocks of life to synthetic pills? We can achieve optimal health when we remove the underlying brain chemical imbalances which lead to the symptoms of moods and depression including insomnia, anxiety, panic reactions, irritability, weight gain, aches and pains, and more.

The good news is that targeted micronutrients and healthy nutrition, along with other holistic methods of healthcare, can reduce or eliminate moods and depression, naturally.

BOOK
The Real Cause and Solution for Alcohol Addiction
The NEW Alcoholism Story
by Suka Chapel-Horst, RN, PhD, QMHP, CPLT

Alcohol addiction is caused by an inherited and genetically caused imbalance of brain chemistry. It's not caused by a character defect, a moral shortcoming, or by a lack of will power.

Neuroscience and biochemistry have proven, once and for all, that all addictions are biochemically caused. It's time to give up shame, blame, and guilt for a disorder that is biochemically caused.

When dysfunctional brain chemistry is restored to normal, relapse and dry-drunk symptoms are rare. Learn how imbalanced brain chemistry leads to alcoholism and discover the recovery method that has the highest long-term relapse-free recovery rate.

BOOK
Cannabinoids – The Hundredth Monkey Cure
by Suka Chapel-Horst, RN, PhD, QMHP, CPLT

The human body naturally produces cannabis-like chemicals that keep all body systems in balance. This internal cannabinoid system may be the most important health discovery of recent years. THC, CBN, and CBD from the cannabis sativa plant mimic our internal chemicals and work to improve our overall health. Cannabidiol, or CBD, cures or relieves symptoms of over 100 disorders. ...and it's legal everywhere because it doesn't have the psycho-active ingredient, THC.

Want better natural solutions for your health concerns? This DVD shows how to change brain chemistry and improve your life by using Cannabidiol (CBD), amino acids, neuronutrients, nutrition, exercise, and chronic stress reducers. Say goodbye to anxiety, stress, depression, insomnia, pain, physical disorders, and much more.

BOOK
The Gift – A Sound Mind for Life
by Suka Chapel-Horst, RN, PhD, QMHP, CPLT

How to increase mental focus, improve memory, and prevent or delay Alzheimer's. Find out about the effects of stress and how to minimize it in order to prolong health and quality life. The DVD includes biochemical, nutritional, physical, emotional, and mental resources to minimize and delay the effects of aging. This is valuable information for any age.
BOOK

PTSD – Post-Traumatic Stress Disorder
Alternative Resources for Recovery
by Suka Chapel-Horst, RN, PhD, QMHP, CPLT

Medications have long term, harmful side effects, including addiction, and traditional counseling methods are often only partially effective.

There are two underlying causes of PTSD. 1) Biochemical deficiencies, or brain chemistry imbalances, and 2) underlying, UNCONSCIOUS, unresolved trauma which occurred PRIOR to the known trauma-experience that *appears* to be the cause of PTSD. These unconscious memories are called *source trauma.*

Addressing biochemical, nutritional, brain wave state, and bioenergy fields is a necessary component to recovery, including the clearing of destructive cellular memories using the latest science of energy psychology.

Uncovering and resolving hidden source trauma, the underlying cause of PTSD, is accomplished with *Integrative Memory Therapy*®. (See page 31.)

These books and DVDs can be ordered through:
www.IMRIWellness.org
www.AriseAlcoholRecovery.com
Or by calling: 417-380-3254

Suka Chapel-Horst

www.ingramcontent.com/pod-product-compliance
Lightning Source LLC
Chambersburg PA
CBHW070341290526
45791CB00003B/1427